THE
ENEMY
WITHIN

MY JOURNEY BATTLING MULTIPLE SCLEROSIS

THE
ENEMY
WITHIN

MY JOURNEY BATTLING
MULTIPLE SCLEROSIS

By

ERIC GAITHO

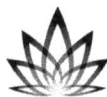

CONSCIOUS CARE PUBLISHING PTY LTD

THE ENEMY WITHIN

MY JOURNEY BATTLING MULTIPLE SCLEROSIS

Copyright © 2021 by Eric Gaitho. All rights reserved.

First Published 2021 by: Conscious Care Publishing Pty Ltd
PO Box 776, Rockingham, WA 6968, Australia
www.consciouscarepublishing.com

First Edition printed December 2021.

National Library of Australia Cataloguing-in-Publication entry:
Author: Gaitho, Eric
The Enemy Within / by Eric Gaitho
ISBN 9780645089233 (Paperback)
ISBN 9780645089240 (ePub)
Angela MacDonald, Editor

Printed by Lightning Source
Typeset & cover design by Conscious Care Publishing Pty Ltd

ISBN: 978-0-6450892-3-3

To my dear wife Jane and baby Chege,

This is for you.

ACKNOWLEDGEMENTS

I cannot thank my dear family and friends enough for being my pillar of hope and support. To all the doctors in Australia and China, physiotherapists, personal trainers, counsellors, dieticians, naturopaths, MS associations, MS warriors and MS researchers I have met over the years since my diagnosis, may you continue to carry your banners high and continue to help us fight this condition.

PREFACE

'...Then it happened. It was a Wednesday morning. I had a 7 a.m. shift start. I woke up fine. I prepared to go to the office fine. I drove to work fine and went to sign in and pretty much start my shift fine. The Australian weather can get rather cheeky, especially during season change from summer to autumn. Out of nowhere, the skies decided to wet the ground, and there was a flash rain. Believe me that is what it was. First, there was sun and clear blue skies. A few minutes later, rain and a clear blue sky in no time after that. During this 'rain', I wanted to run straight to the office, but then all hell broke loose. I could not run. I had the plan of running to shelter from the rain, but my legs did not acknowledge the command. I was freaking out at this point. I had to open another door, unfortunately setting off several alarms, for me to be able to gain access to the shopping centre....'

ABOUT THE AUTHOR

Since a young age, Eric was not 'school-inclined', but this was not the case a few years later when he graduated with a degree in Law and soon after, a master's degree in the same field from an Australian University. Right after his graduation, he was diagnosed with Multiple Sclerosis, which is still an incurable, degenerative condition. Eric was informed that he could not pursue a legal career because of the potential of work-related stress, of which he agreed. Having been advised to turn away from a career that he had dedicated six years of study for, it was no surprise that he was worried of his mental health. In 2016, Eric and his then girlfriend (now wife) travelled to China for a Stem Cell treatment. The results were promising at the onset, and he was drug free for months.

Later that same year, Eric started feeling unwell again and, having gone through the symptoms a few years earlier, visited the neurologist only to be told that the condition had shown activity in the scans that had been ordered. He was put back on medication which he still receives every six weeks. In 2017 he trained to be a travel agent and the following year he opened a travel business that he operated from home after realising how difficult it was to find employment that would accommodate his physical demands. Eric's plan for his business was to have broken even in two years. This did not eventuate as a global pandemic forced him to close the business in 2020. Refusing to let this stop him, he is currently studying a master's degree in counselling. Eric is an advocate for the promotion of men's mental health which he thinks is ignored.

This book is meant to show people that life may deal cards to a person that will be unexpected, but we can all rise above such challenges.

Eric has changed his career three times in less than 10 years due to circumstances beyond his control. Now with a wife and son, he hopes that is his final career change.

CONTENTS

A lot of people commend me for being strong, fearless, and brave. According to them, instead of complaining when my health is such a big challenge to me, I always find a reason to smile. One of my best sayings to date is:

'There are no great men, just great challenges ordinary men like you and I must face.'

This is, and will always remain, my position. I did not choose this condition. I am not sure of the opposite, though.

What God gifted me with, and I plan to use it against this health challenge, is the will to fight and the thirst to win. Life may seem to have blindsided me but once is enough if you ask me. From here on, it is on.

With God by my side and my family and friends in my corner for support, let's do this.

Eric Gaitho

CHAPTER 1

HOW THE STORY BEGAN

I had a great upbringing. I was introduced to this beautiful world on 24th February to a lovely couple, Esther Gaitho and Francis Gaitho, and the little Wendy Gaitho. After two years, my younger brother, Martin, was born, and that was my family. I say 'was' because the family is growing. My sister is now married with two adorable kids plus my in-law family, and I am married with a gorgeous baby boy and adding my wife's family to my family. My brother has yet to add to this number, and best of all, we are not done yet.

I had a very active childhood. My siblings, cousins, and family friends made it more interesting with consequences that have been denied, vehemently, by the perpetrators (I am serious. Any punishment and whatever followed are unequivocally refuted by my mom and all involved parties. I find it funny how they refuse what we 'claim' but defend their actions by asking a very suggestive question. They always ask, 'if you lot were not whooped, you would not be where you are right now, would you?' Well, I guess we will never find out.) True story, we were once at my cousin's place comparing notes of what disciplinary actions had been served on us when we were younger. One of our friends from Ireland was around. After we finished exchanging our experiences, he looked at us with a worried look, and he asked how it was that we had no mental breakdown when we were young. The answer, we did not have that option. For this reason, the people who maintain that disciplining a child causes mental health issues, well, let me set the record straight, it does not. I know many 'level-headed' people who would be in a mental health asylum if it did, including myself.

Most days were spent outdoors. Tree climbing, silly games, swimming in rivers (risky, but we were young, and what was considered fun was not safe). We only went back into the house for lunch, then we went back outside playing until around 5:30 p.m. because we had specific instructions to be back home before sunset. Oh, and no reporting. If one of you tripped the other or caused another to get hurt, mask the hurt or injury because we were punished as a group.

My parents decided to send me to school a year earlier than expected, and it was fantastic (My family members will laugh at that statement because I skipped school on day 1 and again a couple of years later. Both times in dramatic fashion. Let's just say I was not very fond of school). My siblings and I attended the same school. We had two choices of us getting there, 1) my mum drops us off as she heads to work, which means we get to school very early, or 2) we walk there with our friends and get there just before class. We were fortunate that the school we attended was close by, and it always was an exciting stroll. In 1997, our dad died. My sister and I were old enough to understand the gravity of what had happened, but our younger brother, not so much.

School was an experience for us all. There are certain times that we were and in the same school with one or the other. This was primarily with my brother, who used to swing based on my sister's performance, or myself, mainly my sister, who was more academically inclined. My career line, on the other hand, speaks very differently about this factor. A lawyer who hated school.

High school. The school I started my first year of high school in was the same school I finished in four years later. This was the same case with my sister. Our younger brother, on the other hand, let us just say he wanted to experience it from different schools. Hey, I'm trying to use positive wording here. We were done with high school, and we were all in university. I did my undergraduate in West Africa. To be more specific, in Ghana, because I had ended up becoming a party maniac, and my mom knew I would not study if the decision were left to me. Two of my friends and I decided to make sure we enjoyed our youth and that we did. Years later, I can publicly admit that it was the best decision ever. One of us became a top officer in the armed forces, the other is an advocate in Kenya. My mom would be the best person to ask the story behind the choice of Ghana. I initially considered it treachery owing to several facts that I thought were borderline illegal. However, it was a decision that had to be made, and we were immature and young to be burdened by such significant decisions. All that aside, I graduated with a Bachelor of Laws degree in 2010. For a person who was not fond of school and education/authority, this was a miracle. My sister always remembers my mom crying through the ceremony during my graduation because she was still in disbelief that I, Eric, was graduating with a degree in Law. She had only wished for such a day.

After my graduation, I went back to Kenya to apply my degree in the legal field. During this period, I met with more friends and new opportunities. I was getting frustrated with trying to make ends meet. Not that I had very many obligations. It is just that I had a false belief that with a law degree, life would be smooth, i.e., find a job, and life would work its magic from there. Lies. I ended up going down an unfortunate road of alcohol dependency. This was the first time that I believe I battled depression. Now I can say that rather than saying I was just 'acting up.' I felt like a let-down to myself, my mom, my siblings, and anyone who expected the best from me. To get this under control, I visited my mom. She worked in war-torn Liberia, and we all thought seeing what she did would bring things back into perspective again. It worked.

I was shocked to see the life war could bring. There were no buildings, no electricity, no roads. It was just a sad state. For electricity, the whole country ran on generators that would be put on for an hour in the morning and during lunchtime and again in the evening for four to five hours. The landlord dictated the exact time to schedule this. My mom used to go to work during the day, and I spent my days reading books, going around the town, and volunteering with some Non-government organisations. What I experienced cannot be described in words. It made me appreciate the peace that my country enjoyed. It was hard to believe that my mom and her team had come to that country just after the civil war. This was years later, and I could feel and see the destruction that had been caused. I knew my mom worked in countries recovering from war but knowing and experiencing are very different. I was literally in the eye of the storm. One of my friends in university feared loud bangs because of what he had experienced in his mother country when he was younger. He is from Sierra Leone. Now I knew why. If that is the effect of war, I hope everyone prays never to experience it. To put my experience into words is challenging enough. I had attended a meeting where a child's experience of the civil war was more than anybody could handle. ANYBODY. This child had been drugged and forced to kill his family members. How will that child live with themselves? I thought what I saw in movies was a lie. It was not.

I had seen the lowest side of life. Liberia was a lesson that hit home. When I went back home, I planned on changing my ways and making the best of the situation that I was in. I started a business with a few friends, but it did not survive for long. I have never forgiven myself for that. Young and dumb. That is what it was. No excuses. We had not been conned any money. Nothing of that nature. We used to party hard after a job, and instead of re-investing

our cash, we wasted it on parties and having a good time. And fun
we had.

CHAPTER 2

KNOCK, KNOCK?

I then moved to Australia to pursue a Master of Laws degree. When studying my undergraduate, I enjoyed 'criminal law' as a unit. So, I was not surprised when I did more 'criminal justice' courses when studying for my Masters's degree. I had come to Australia intending to study environmental law, but curiosity got the best of me. In university, I undertook a unit on environmental law. I had fantastic lecturers, but the content was not something I would have wanted to practice long-term. Then I took a course on criminal justice, and I was sold. I knew I was going to master in that field. There was the study of human behaviour, and this was too enticing. At the end of it all, I was even more curious about the thinking of criminals. What brought about this 'bad' nature?

What made it tick? Could it be controlled, and if so, how? I learned of actions that could reduce the repetition of criminal behaviour, and how the criminal justice system could achieve some of these results, et cetera. There was much reading involved, but it was exciting.

My transition from Ghana to Kenya to Australia was smooth. In a nutshell, Ghanaians are amicable people. True story, on my first day in university, one of my roommates and I were going around the university knowing the place when some guy who had only seen me at the law faculty during registration drove next to us and offered to take us around the university grounds to show us where the essential services were located. In my country of origin, this offer was to be followed by the question, 'say what now?'. We are very cautious people. I reluctantly got in the car, and he did exactly that. After a brief tour of the campus, he gave us his number if we got stranded and needed some help. He dropped us in front of our hostel and bid us farewell. Ghana was my home for the next four years. I used to visit Kenya during semester breaks, but my home was Ghana.

Then I moved to Australia. Being a guy from Nairobi, Kenya, West Africa was the height of 'hot' in my books. Forget what you may have heard from international media about Africa being a sweltering place. It is not. One, Africa is too big a continent to make such an average assumption on the weather there. Two, Kenya has a very vast area that having one kind of temperature trend is, for lack of a better word, impossible. This is pretty much about most, if not all, African states. Oh, and finally, not all Kenyans can run. I cannot stress this enough. Anyway, I thought I had experienced 'HOT' but boy was I wrong. To make things worse, I got to Australia on that extra day of the year, i.e., 29th February. When I left the airport building, I almost went back in to board a flight back to where I had come from. As in, it was disgustingly hot. Then my sister and brother-in-law said that was just the tip of the iceberg. I thought they were joking. They were not.

I started my university, and all was a breeze. It was fun to some extent. Oh, by saying it was all a 'breeze' should not be taken to mean it was easy. Days, and sometimes the best of nights and weekends, were spent in the law library. Yep. More books. After two years, on 8th April 2014, I graduated. My dislike for school and my advancement in the field of 'study' do not go hand in hand. As I was waiting for the graduation date, things started happening that were out of the norm, leading to the unprepared news.

Just as I settled in Australia, living expenses and life, in general, were gradually getting higher. I attempted to get a job, and I was not successful in finding any job to help ease the expenses. One night, I had gone to a nightclub and met a former schoolmate who advised me to get a security licence. I borrowed the money from my sister to pay for the course and underwent the training. After two weeks, I got my licence to be a registered security officer and crowd controller, and a week and a half later, I landed a job. It was such a relief to see an active bank account. I paid my sister back, and I got into security. I retired from the workforce after a few years on the same job and in the same company.

I tend to think being a security officer had less drama than my role as a crowd controller. The people we dealt with in these two roles were the main difference. As a security officer in a shopping centre, I came across retail theft incidents, slip and fall accidents, medical-related incidents, and the likes. Some of them were funny, while some were serious. The most serious was when a customer had a serious accident and unfortunately died a week later. On the flip side, crowd control exposed one to the nasties of drunk, drugged, and rowdy crowds. I remember once Jane, then my girlfriend, dropped me at an event I was to work in. It was an eleven-hour job, and we were meant to provide security to a crowd of 10,000 plus. Piece of cake, I wished. Jane came over to pick me up after my shift, and the look on her face said it all. My shirt was torn, I had lost my neck chain and my wristwatch, and I looked like I had a job of digging up trenches because I was just dirty. I could not wait to get home, have a hot shower, and sleep.

Back to the time when 'stuff' started happening that led to my first retirement from the workforce, I will explain why it was my first. My job, then, required much walking around. I started noticing that I was losing my footing, and I seemed to be bumping into walls on my right as I walked around. Blaming my male nature and my dislike for hospitals, I was concerned but not enough to go and see my GP. I know. One morning I was walking in front of my then supervisor when he approached me asking if my right leg was 'ok.' 'Why?' I asked him. 'Because you seem to be limping. Are you by any chance hurt?' This was news to me as I felt ok. This was just the 'smoke' from a 'fire' I was not ready for. As much as I did not want it to alarm me, my supervisor had a certain 'authority' with his words, and he sounded concerned.

Several days later, I felt a numb sensation in my right leg. This feeling was constant. It was more like the pins and needles that one gets when you wrongly position your leg when you sit down. Now, make that a continuous sensation. Soon after, I started experiencing pain in my left leg. Not the right leg, the left leg. This time around, I felt pain. Still, it was a categorical 'no' to a visit to my GP.

Then it happened. It was a Wednesday morning. I had a 7 a.m. shift start. I woke up fine. I prepared to go to the office fine. I drove to work fine and went to sign in and pretty much start my shift fine. The Australian weather can get rather cheeky, especially during season change from summer to autumn. The skies decided to wet the ground out of nowhere, and there was a 'flash rain'. Believe me that is what it was. First, there was sun and clear blue skies. A few minutes later, rain and a clear blue sky in no time after that. During this 'rain', I had tried to run straight to the office, but all hell broke loose. I could not run. I had the plan of running to shelter from the rain, but my legs did not acknowledge the command. I was freaking out at this point. I had to open another door, unfortunately setting off several alarms, for me to be able to gain access to the shopping centre.

My shift continued and ended without any more drama, but I could not stop wondering what had happened that morning. I kept asking myself, why could I not run? During the day, I had booked an appointment with my GP. Not being able to run had done the trick. I could not deny that something wrong was in motion inside me. Do not get me wrong, I was not a track athlete, so it was not that important that I had to run, but just knowing it was one of the things I could do was, in my mind, a superpower of some form.

After the initial tests, the GP recommended that I arrange an appointment with a neurologist as soon as possible. I joked a lot with my GP, and my bright mind saw this was an excellent time to share a joke. I looked at my GP and told him, 'I hope you now see why I dislike you people (GPs in general). I come to see you, and in turn, you send me to see a neurologist.' He could only afford a smile and with a gaze that screamed concern, 'immediately,' he added. Ok. He referred me to a neurologist whom I called to book an appointment. God was on my side as I could secure an appointment early that afternoon which was possible because I started work at 3 p.m. I insist God intervened because it could have taken months to get an opening for an appointment with a specialist, from what I had heard. I was very fortunate to call immediately after one of his patients called to cancel their appointment. What are the chances?

I was eager to see the neurologist and finally figure out what was cooking. This position is debatable now because the result of this appointment was not what I had expected. Ever. I remember this appointment like it was yesterday. The neurologist had received my presenting symptoms from my GP and knew what he would face when getting to that examination room. He came in. A calm, collected guy. For some reason, I thought he would have this 'serious' kind of look. My bad Dr. G, in case you get to read this. Then he introduced himself and a summary of why my GP had forwarded my case to him. Then came the 'stand on one leg, look there, squeeze my fingers, do you feel the same sensation on both legs and hands?' This physical examination took roughly twenty to thirty minutes.

As he told me the physical test was done, he had a worried stare. When I worked as a lawyer, one of the first things I was taught was to study people's facial expressions, which would assist me when filing an assessment for a potential client. Here was a situation when this lesson was not needed but worthwhile as it was now a habit. He warmed me to the idea of MS. He asked me whether I knew anything about it. 'Nothing. I've just seen an advert for an MS lottery on TV', I replied, being as honest as I could be. 'Go home and have a read, then plan an appointment in a week, and I will answer all your questions then. I'm sure you will have a lot of them.' And with that, he gracefully walked to the door, bid me farewell, and held the door for my exit.

Well, now, aside from getting an awkward, concerned look from a neurologist whom I had never met before, I had homework. My dislike graph was on danger levels concerning the medical fraternity.

I left the doctor's consulting rooms straight to work. I had to get my game-face on as it was one of those nights that was always busy. At 6:00 p.m., we had a team meeting when we got a briefing from my supervisor and manager. The briefing went ok, and it was over in fifteen minutes. Everybody headed out once it was over, and I remained behind to brief my supervisor and manager regarding my neurologist appointment. With a smile and hoping for a positive reaction, my manager enthusiastically asked me what the doctor had said. I replied, 'he said something on the lines of MS. I have another appointment with the guy next week to get a better understanding of the problem.' She gasped.

I guess this is an excellent time to paint a picture of my manager. After many years in the security industry, she was a person who was never shocked about many things that would surprise the ordinary person. And this was something I had had just two years of, and you get to witness the most shocking behaviours and characters. She had years of this under her belt. In short, not a lot shocked J, but this did. Now I was curious. I think I worked my shift wondering what this 'MS' was that seemed to shake J. Thank God that Thursday was smooth sailing with no drama. I was done by 9:00 p.m. and out of the door heading home. I got home, had dinner with Jane, and gave her a summary of my day when we got to bed. She also seemed alarmed that J had gasped when I mentioned 'MS.' We were both too curious, and we quickly checked what Dr. Google had on it. I now understood why the neurologist had said I would have many questions. Why, oh why did we not sleep on it? Why?

I will not lie; that night, I do not think I slept. What had I just read? Oh, by the way, Google should never be used to check on symptoms or anything to do with one's health. General information can be googled like the number of countries globally, but anything to do with one's health, call your GP or your friend in the medical fraternity. I had not read anything positive or hopeful in it. I am sure Jane was in the same boat. I could feel her toss and turn the whole night. When morning came, I was still tired, understandably so. I was short of words to tell Jane. I just wished her a good day ahead as she left for work. I was lucky I never used to work Friday and Saturday. At least it gave me time to 'try' and digest the news. I kept asking myself, 'What did I just read? How can my body be doing this to itself?' I even took time to think of what mistakes I had made to be in my position. Little did I know this was the beginning of an exceedingly long and challenging journey.

I went back to work on Sunday. All seemed normal, but my mind was on overdrive. I could not stop wondering about what Jane and I had read. In a way, I even started blaming myself for living a very 'careless' life before I came to Australia. I was always drinking and smoking. Like, a lot. In a day, I used to drink a substantial amount of alcohol and go through two packets of cigarettes. I kept away from drugs. My phobia for needles somewhat saved my life. I could not even dream of an injection near me. Until today, after years of four-weekly and later six-weekly infusions, I have not gathered enough courage to look at the cannula insertion when they are prepping me for my infusions.

All my life, I had heard that we should aim at having a healthy immune system. Well, never had I thought that that same immune system would end up causing such damage. From the little I had read, MS is when the immune system attacks the nervous system. My body was literally eating itself up, and there was nothing I could do to prevent it. NOTHING. When I was growing up, I had heard of a theory (not confirmed in my books) that wild animals are put down if they come in contact with human flesh because they will develop an urge to have more, leading to more killing.

MS is somewhat the same. Once it attacks the nervous system, it can't get enough. I am now on a six-weekly medication which in essence 'gears down' my immune system to maintain the 'status quo,' so to speak. It used to be every twenty-eight days, but as time goes by and the more stable I become with the dosage, the neurologist I see keeps updating it.

I only had one question for the neurologist a week later. 'You want to tell me that my body is doing this to itself?' was the question I posed to the neurologist. What is funny is that I knew the answer was a simple 'YES,' but it became real when it came from the doctor. Dr. G made the dreaded, unsurprising news on my second appointment with him. Since my first appointment, I think I had a medical test carried out daily during my week. 'All the tests indicate you have Multiple Sclerosis'. Yep. Those words still hurt to this day. I can remember the doctor giving me instructions on ways to cope with this news. Ok. Truth be told, I could see his mouth moving, but that was it. I did not hear any words. Call it shock or whatever.

I drove straight home. I was somewhat happy. Not because of the diagnosis but at least the problems I was having had an answer. Dealing with the answer is another thing altogether. I then got ready for work. Yes. I needed the distraction, and a Thursday night shift would do the trick. My manager made sure I worked a three-hour shift. Somehow, she knew I needed to get my mind away from the news. My whole team synced on that fact. To this day, I will forever be grateful to each of them for knowing I had received disturbing information, masking it, and making me as comfortable as they could.

To be honest, I had not seen this coming.

CHAPTER 3

MULTIPLE SCLEROSIS (MS) DEFINED

Being someone who hates needles, I never thought they would be a frequent companion just before and after my diagnosis. From my first neurologist appointment to the time I received the diagnosis, the number of hospital visits was extreme. Something was being done every day, and sometimes more than one test was being carried out. I was fortunate my workplace was accommodating and quite flexible with my shifts. There are very many nurses in Western Australia, and if you get to a point where they know you by name, my friend, you are becoming a regular. That was me. My hands made one think had a substance abuse habit because of the multiple injection marks. Dr. G referred me to two other neurologists for a second and third opinion. This was to satisfy his curiosity that what he had diagnosed as MS was precisely that. According to Dr. G, I did not 'qualify' for MS. This was a period that I came to know a lot about what was wrong with me. As in health-wise. Sanity-wise, debatable. All the tests I did with Dr. G, I did with Dr. L and Dr. B. Bloodwork, MRI scans, physical examinations, lumbar punctures. The whole thing.

I think it is high time I mention the types of MS. There are four types of MS (unless this count has changed, which will not be surprising considering the medical advancements and research that is ongoing). I will mention them in order of severity. First is Clinically Isolated Syndrome (CIS), where a person may suffer 'MS-like' symptoms, but it does not develop into MS. The second is Relapsing-Remitting MS (RRMS). This is the most common form of the condition, with approximately 85% of people who receive an MS diagnosis being diagnosed with RRMS. The sufferer will experience attacks of new and/or increased symptoms (relapses), followed by partial or complete recovery (remission). I was diagnosed with RRMS and to best explain the temporary nature and permanency of some symptoms, I will use my case as an example. After diagnosis, I lost the ability to write and drive a car, but I can now write and drive ok, but I'm still trying to shake off using a walking stick years later. Next is Secondary Progressive MS (SPMS), which is characterised by worsening neurological function. To note here is that RRMS can progress to SPMS, but one can also receive a diagnosis of SPMS, and the symptoms will be worse than that of someone who gets an RRMS diagnosis. Finally, we have Primary Progressive MS (PPMS). Approximately 10% of people diagnosed with MS are diagnosed with PPMS, which is characterised by worsening neurological function from the onset without relapse or remission.

Researchers have come up with a list of factors that might cause MS or 'increase' someone's likelihood of receiving an MS diagnosis. Yes. There is such a 'qualification' list that indicated that I was not a candidate. Disclaimer, I am not medically trained, so you can add to the list below if you know of more factors. First, heredity. Ok. This is where I had to dig deep into my family linage. Luckily, my brother had worked on our family tree not too long before, and there was no indication of any form of MS within the family. That was an easy one to cross off the list. The second factor was injury. This was very broad considering my lifestyle in my teen years, where everything could be attempted. In high school, I delved into the fantastic game of rugby. Injuries were unavoidable, and to find out they were not the cause of the MS, interesting is an understatement. I had to undergo a lumbar puncture to confirm this. This is one of those medical procedures that I will never be a fan of. If anyone is reading this and hates the sight of an injection, be warned. For a lumbar puncture to occur, the guy (I have never known their medical name. I dislike the procedure that much) doing it sticks a needle in your spine to get a sample of someone's 'spinal fluid.' This fluid undergoes several tests, and the results help the doctors to rule out injury. Yeah. It is one of those procedures. To date, I have had five of them. Yep. Then it gets vaguer. The third is environmental factors. I received the diagnosis in 2014, but to date, I have no clue what this is. Under this factor, a person's environment is considered the reason behind the MS. How? Only MS researchers can help you out here.

Countries further from the equator have more people diagnosed with the condition. An example, New Zealand will have more cases of MS than Australia. Also, MS sufferers have a deficiency of vitamin D, which is absorbed primarily from the sun. Another detail with my case that made it peculiar was that I had migrated from Kenya, literally at the equator. I was not supposed to have any deficiency of vitamin D. I had spent almost my whole life in Kenya. I went to Ghana during my campus years, which is hotter than Kenya, and the sun was never an issue. Believe me. Despite these facts, my tests showed a deficiency in vitamin D. Also, for close to two years, I had minimal contact with the sun as I worked the night shift and I was asleep during the day. I was happy about this, initially, because the Australian sun was like no other. If the sun comes into contact with your bare skin in Kenya and Ghana, meaning your arms, legs, and neck, you break a sweat. Your body gets hot. In Australia, the sun touches any part of your skin, you itch. Yes. Itch. I just avoided it. The other part of environmental factors is diet. Anything under this, I have come across it mainly through my dietician and a lot of reading.

The next three factors made me a more 'unlikely candidate'. These, I believe, were pretty much what pushed the doctors to carry out more tests on me. I found it rather amusing that there may be people who are more susceptible to such a condition. Sad even. The first was age. A diagnosis of MS is likely to be made for someone in their mid-forties and above. I was twenty-eight. With time, I came to question this rationale, especially when I heard of someone as young as nine who was an MS warrior. Then comes sex. The ratio of men to women with the condition is 1:3. This I have taken with a pinch of salt. I am yet to be convinced. Lastly is race. Black people are rarely diagnosed with MS. As I have previously indicated, one of the primary deficiencies with people diagnosed with MS is low vitamin D. Considering most African kids spend most of their time playing outside, they rarely suffer a low vitamin D count. I was once in an Uber with a young man from the northern parts of Kenya who was shocked that we had extremely different vitamin D levels coming from the same country. He had been informed that his vitamin D levels were the highest his GP had ever come across. My childhood, in a few words, unless the rain stopped me from going out and the arse whooping that would follow my coming home with muddy clothing, I woke up, had my breakfast, went out to play until it was lunchtime, came home for lunch, then left to go continue playing until the sun went down. I am sure I did this all day, every day. When I grew older and my level of play had decreased, I enjoyed walking around campus. Ok. It also saved me money. If my memory serves me right, I only had a disconnect with the sun when I came to Australia. I can attribute this to two main reasons: the sun was ridiculously hot and working night shifts. These seemed to be challenging factors to the doctors because they maintained I had spent just over two years in Australia, which was a noticeably short period, but the results showed a problem.

In my opinion, the above summary of what MS is, the types of MS, and what causes MS is just my understanding. I am sure there might be issues a medical mind might think I have skipped, but I am trying to make it as simple as possible to understand. I am trying to avoid repeating my experience with encountering a condition I knew nothing of and bombarding myself with all this information in one go.

It took a lot of self-conversations to convince myself that this was happening. I thanked God whatever was happening did not happen when I was working night shifts. At least during the day, I had a team of workmates who would help if stuff was to go wrong. Stuff going wrong on specific jobs might be considered rare, but that is the job in security. One minute all is breezy, and the next minute, all hell breaks loose. That was us. Clearly, I was on the clock.

My then manager came up with an idea that would significantly reduce my time on the floor and benefit the job. I was in the security office through my shift doing 'clerical' jobs and CCTV surveillance. This increased the manning hours on the floor and reduced the amount of time spent by security personnel in the security office. Let us just say it was a terrific band-aid solution for a situation we had not seen coming. I was now working six hours a day from Monday to Friday. This was an ok change from night-shift work

It was relaxing going around the shopping centre on a scooter, but I was sad all at the same time. I could not believe how fast things were happening, for example, running one day and on a scooter the next. And just like that, I slowly went into a drinking habit. Not at work. No. But after. I would use alcohol to drown my sorrows and sleep, waiting for the next day and doing it all over again. Having been in a drinking habit before, I thought I would be stronger, but it won. Again.

CHAPTER 4

THE STAGES OF GRIEF

At that moment, I did not put too much thought into it, but when I came to give it some thought later, I realised I was going through what is better known as 'Stages of Grief'. Denial, anger, bargaining, depression, and acceptance. What I found interesting with this 'theory', if I may call it that, is the simple fact that what I went through was exactly as they were outlined. Each stage with its demons and struggles, but I covered all five stages. I will describe each with as much accuracy and truth as I can.

Denial. It was tricky because I had no idea what I had and what I could potentially face in the future. What made me fear the 'unknown' was the concern in my then GP's voice and my manager, who simply gasped when she heard the words 'MS' come out of my mouth. Here I was about to graduate. I had considered myself to be at the prime of my life, plans of a bright future were playing vividly in my mind, a girlfriend who I planned to propose to and graduating to pursue a career I had only dreamt of and spent the last six years studying to be good at. In short, I thought I was almost there. Then suddenly MS. 'What am I facing?' 'What is going on?' 'I was so close. Why now?' 'This can't be happening.' Yeah. This was me. My mind was like a trivia show. Question after question. Too close yet too far. I come from a Christian family, I was brought up a Christian, and I swore to never ask, 'Why me God?' That I did not bring myself to ask. I think it is the only question I have never asked. My faith will never let me.

One day I am healthy and chasing after troubled individuals, and the next thing I know, I'm on a scooter cruising the mall. It was 'awkward,' to say the least. It was hard for me to believe that this was happening. Have you ever watched an interesting movie, and you miss a very crucial part, and you press the pause button and the rewind button to where you think it happened? This was me, and the movie was my life. I pressed the pause and the rewind button on my life, trying to figure out when MS happened. This was not an easy task because I had had a rather interesting life. To briefly describe what I am talking about, think of anything and assume I had done it, apart from two things. I never have, and in that case, never will inject myself. NEVER. So, any drugs or whatever crazy thing that involves injecting myself, never done. Never will. The last activity I ever did that involved blood; I was still a child who loved to chew on carrots. I had seen my mom and nanny peel them and thought it was a good idea to do so. Child + knife + inexperience = disaster. I almost sliced my finger off. Since then, I believe my blood is supposed to remain in my body. Sharp things, i.e., knives and needles, should be handled by professionals.

Blood and I can be equated to oil and water. They do not mix. My mom always reminded me of a time in my childhood when I saw blood and believed I would die. Yep. DYING. Even if it was a splinter. To me, blood = death. No two ways about it. I thought this was over when I was older, but I was so wrong. I was about nineteen years old when I went for major dental surgery; I did everything to avoid seeing the massive injection that would go into my mouth to administer the numbing medication. Everything was going ok until I felt some liquid droplets on my arm. 'Sorry about that, just a bit of blood, but everything else is good', the dentist says. I, on the other hand, heard 'blood', and that was it. I started shaking uncontrollably, and the dentist had to stop operating first until I relaxed for him to finish up. I went home after the procedure, and the dentist asked why the convulsions during a follow-up session. 'Blood,' I told him. Just the mention of it was enough.

When I got to Australia, my mom had her concerns when she heard I could be in a situation where I would be forced to administer first aid, but I never had a problem dealing with blood during my work. I seemed to be ok with someone else's blood, but I can't watch medical TV programs that show blood.

When I got the diagnosis, 'denial' was fed by the fact that I could not do what I could do a few days before. I was not worried about my health, education, health cover, job security, and all that.

Just the fact that I could not be my old self anymore. Not that I was always proud of the life I had lived in my youth and not that I was disappointed in it either or in any way regretted it. On this issue, one belief I stick by is that 'One is allowed to recognize that a decision was made, but they should not regret it'. I always considered regret as another way of living in the past, and unfortunately, we do not have the luxury of time to do that. A good or a wrong decision has been made, and nothing could be said or done to better the outcome.

At the back of my mind, despite all that was happening, I kept telling myself, 'This can't be it'. I had multiple blood tests, medical examinations, and all, trying to figure out what was happening to me. I think it was the shock of all that was happening, but I could not accept whatever was happening. 'This can't be me', 'I have just finished my Master's degree', 'I have many dreams and aspirations', 'Where might I have messed up?' 'How did this creep up without any detection?' My mind never stopped questioning everything.

It was quite a coincidence that my mom was going through her health challenge back in Kenya. She was fine one day, and the next, she was not. Cancer had decided to give her a run for her money. She won. This gave me some form of consolation because it simply proved that bad luck was not on my plate, and I am sure it somehow gave my mom another reason to fight harder because I am afraid that if she had given up or if Cancer won, it would have broken me. Nowadays, I sit around with my mom and say how 'we' survived while silently one is telling the other, 'you gave me the strength to give my all'.

Another reality I was struggling with was the change of roles in our relationship. As I grew up, I had learned that it was the duty of the man to fend for his family. I had received a diagnosis that would change all that. I knew that I would end up spending a lot of downtime at home, and Jane would be the one going to work. It was a very foreign concept to me, but it was the reality. There would come a time when I could not go to work, and the best I could do was make sure I saw the end of the day. I also knew that when the time came when we would start a family, I would be a stay home dad. This was new territory to me. Since I was young, my siblings and I spent most of our time with our mom while my dad was away for work duties. Not that I'm complaining, but this is what I knew was the norm, which would not be so. This also built up a worry regarding finances. Yes, we had been taught about saving for a 'rainy day', but this was not a day. It was an 'until death do we part' kind of deal from what I had read. To me, that means that whatever finances I had saved would run out at some point. Right now, I look back and see how mentally unhealthy that period was.

Anger was stage two. In case you are wondering, I used to walk around like a ticking bomb. Something small would set me off. You did not have to punch me to expect a reaction. Any wrong move at the wrong time (which was always) would do the trick, and considering the job I was in, I prayed for God to give me strength to face each day as it came and avoid unnecessary rage issues. I expected a different set of challenges each day, but I had a great team behind me.

At home, it was not that easy. Growing up without a father had changed me into a very secretive person. I never spoke about what was bugging me, if ever something was. I strongly think this had influenced my choice of career. Issues of 'privacy' and 'confidentiality' never were a problem to me. Now here I was with a huge health problem, a very wonderful lady as a partner, random rage issues, not being able to share though my dear Jane could notice something was wrong with me, let's just say I was a mess.

'I'm ok' was a statement not new to Jane. I have always been a bad sleeper, and I could only afford to shut my eyes for a couple of hours. It hurt me because every time I woke up at night and wanted to scream, I could not. Not at anything specific. I constantly had the feeling of carrying all the world's problems on my shoulders. Some Hercules business. I never knew how it felt like to feel so helpless that you just sit and stare.

I always felt the need to just talk to Jane, but this never eventuated. There was this one time that I thought maybe crying would help. I tried. I did. Nothing. Have you ever concentrated on getting some tears rolling down to no avail? It is funny but serious at the same time. I did not want to see my face at that moment. I knew I was angry, but I had no outlet. Now I have a punching bag in my home gym and a lot of weights to help me out, but I did not have them then. And off-loading my frustrations on my dear Jane would be unfair. She had been there for me, and hurting her was something I knew was to be avoided at whatever cost. I knew it was not easy on her. Here she was with this dude she had made plans with, and all of a sudden, a health challenge comes to interrupt everything. Not just a health challenge but a life-long condition.

Then came a stage which was a bit of misplaced fun. Bargaining. This, to me, was the most expensive and full of a lot of guesswork. I know this was not the setting for guesswork, but I decided to join the bandwagon now that professionals in the medical fraternity, who I had expected to know what was wrong, seemed to be in the dark too. Do not get me wrong; these guys are dope. I might be taking a very wild guess here, but since my first brush with MS, most of the people I have dealt with are great, but my question of 'what exactly is MS and where does it come from?' is yet to be answered.

I say most expensive because I ended up trying a lot to 'correct' any damage I might have caused my body for it to rebel the way it did. I had read somewhere that I needed to go gluten-free. I tried. Really tried. Summary, I failed. The reason, yuk. The food was so expensive and tasted ... (No words). On to the next one. Drink this, eat that, do not drink this, do not eat that. It never stopped, and the theories never stopped coming. This went on for months. Finally, I had to just drop everything. It had become an obsession. I am sure I checked on ways someone could improve their health if they smoked and drank a lot of alcohol in the past. Theories over theories. At the time, I thought one good deed to my body would correct it all. Boy was I wrong. Every time I tried something, and I saw no results, I got irritated for a while, and soon I was back on the search again. I tried a lot of stuff. And to make matters worse, my understanding of 'MS' was not great. I treated it like I would a cold. I thought if I drank a. b. c, I would wake up feeling better. Yeah. My understanding was on those lines. Now I know more, and I am more informed.

Stage four, depression. This was to be the elephant in the room for my journey. I wish my understanding and appreciation of being mentally healthy that I have now was in my emotional arsenal then. I had to battle thought of suicide and self-harm constantly. And by constantly, I mean CONSTANTLY. Non-stop. Night and day. As you go to sleep and as you wake up. Over and over and over. I had to be on my toes with it. I was afraid of what I would do if I let the thoughts take over. I had to force myself to get out of bed at times. It was a scary time. I love cooking, and I love the kitchen, but for this period, I hated it. I FEARED it. Blades, glass objects, the ease of having an 'accident'. It was too much for me. The one place I could relax and enjoy some 'me' time had turned into the place I feared the most. It got to a point where I did not eat, I stayed thirsty, I kept away from the kitchen at all costs.

One day I remember vividly, because I have wanted to forget it so much, was a day I had decided to ignore my hesitations and go into the kitchen to wash some fruit. I picked up the fruit and walked to the kitchen sink. I turned on the water, and as I washed the fruit, I saw a knife. It was as if it was speaking to me, asking me to pick it up. My hands were shaking at this point. I put down the fruit. I pick the knife up and just run my finger across the blade. Thank God I hate pain because when I felt a sharp prick on my finger, I quickly dropped the knife.

Australia is a country that is keen on mental health wellbeing, and after any distressing news broadcasts, a phone number is displayed that one can call to speak to a counsellor. Lifeline, they call themselves. I had saved the number on my phone for a rainy day. This was not a rainy day, it was a storm, and one of the saddest parts was that I did not open up to anybody about my fears and frustrations. Not that I did not have people to speak to. I had plenty of people to open up to but talking about emotional baggage was not a strength I had. This is the first time I have given that story. Only three people knew about it. God, the counsellor who picked up that call on that day, and myself. Sometimes I would just be in bed, admiring the ceiling, and thoughts of painless ways of 'erasing' myself would creep in. They made me quite uneasy because I was meant to relax, possibly meditate, but most of the time I tried, there they would go again. I would be driving, and thoughts of 'how to fake an accident' would come. I would go past a pharmacy, there they would go again, trying to think of which medications I could buy without raising eyebrows to help with my plan. Keeping my thoughts straight was a full-time job but, I had to 'be a man' and 'deal with it'. Now I know better. Me wanting to maintain the whole 'cool, easy going' persona nearly cost me my life. I thank God I did not succumb to those dark voices.

Sorry to say but, to me, this is where society went wrong. Yes, men have a significant role in society. Yes, men are the backbone of a family and take it from me; that is something we do not take lightly, but as my wife puts it, I am the head of our family, but she is the neck that controls the head. Men are supposed to be 'macho,' but they do crack. We will survive a lot, but that does not make us supernatural. We will be strong for the sake of our families, but we have to 'check' ourselves. We must be watchful of our mental state.

We will be strong, but my wife, family, or friends must ensure I do not overestimate my strength because it is very possible. Look at most suicides; most people will be like, ' they were constantly laughing or that they did not look like they had anything bothering them.' Unfortunately, that is it. Mental health challenges are a silent killer. One looks good today, and the next thing, they are no more. People are left wondering how it happened. 'They seemed ok', most will say. I once read somewhere that 'we can fake a smile, but we cannot fake depression'.

As for me, a dear friend of mine knew that news of a medical condition such as MS would be devastating news to bear on any person. I withdrew from many activities that required people's participation, but my guardian angel used to pass by our house to 'check' on how I was doing. He would swing by and request (I am being courteous) that we step out for a drink. I lived near an Irish pub, and this was easy to plan. It seems like a small act, but it made a big difference to me. This was an hour or two away from my worries. Away from disturbing thoughts. Away from the disastrous reality of MS. We would have a silly conversation going. We knew each other from way back, and we would not lack something to talk about. He might not know it yet (I doubt it), but he was my saving grace. I will forever be grateful, and I will never forget what this individual did for me. I mean that. He is our son's godfather. Thank you, Sam (he said I should address him as Sir, Your Highness, blah, blah, blah … when I mention him here).

Finally, the crème de la crème, acceptance. The most difficult but the most beneficial of the five steps. The most difficult because it was a reality I was not ready to accept. The most helpful because accepting the change of the situation was healthy for my mental state, which was less tasking to the body. I had to accept that not so long ago, I could do stuff that was now impossible, and by saying this, I mean it. One day I could run; the next, I could not. One day I could write (legible or otherwise is another thing) the next, even writing my name was a problem. One day I could stroll down the street; the next, I had to have the help of a walking stick. One day I could drive; the next, I could not. I was fortunate all the above happened on different occasions.

Allow me to digress and explain the effects of MS. Firstly, what makes it hard for a treatment to be developed, in my opinion, is that MS affects people differently. There are some similarities in the symptoms; for example, all the MS warriors I have met have a low vitamin D count. Effects are rather diverse. I know some MS warriors in wheelchairs. Others cannot use their hands. Others cannot see. Others cannot swallow. Others cannot talk. If you ask me, this one fact has brought about one of the most significant mis-understandings of this condition.

After my diagnosis, I considered it somewhat misguided when I heard specific comments coming my way when some people learned I had MS. 'Oh, but you don't look sick' or 'Why are you not in a wheelchair?' or 'Are you drunk this time of the morning?' I will answer these questions one at a time. Unlike other conditions, I do not look sick because MS affects people on the inside more, and I do not think there is a 'look' when MS is at play. Why am I not in a wheelchair? Because MS has not affected my walking to the extent of needing one. Not every MS warrior is in a wheelchair. Why do I seem drunk early in the morning? I am sure your perception would be the same if you stood by my bed when I woke up. Stability, being one of my main challenges, makes me stagger almost everywhere.

I refer to MS patients as 'warriors' because that is what they are. MS is a battle, and you must go at it guns blazing. It is an all-out war. It will have no mercy on the warrior; hence it requires none. Thus, the use of the prefix 'warrior'.

After the stem cell treatment, I realised my endurance when exercising had improved, and I could comfortably workout as long as I had a fan on near my workout station to help keep cool. I took advantage of this, and I started going for physio every week and built up a home gym which was helpful when driving became an issue. This action has changed the trajectory of how MS has affected me. People have noticed improvements, and this has brought about looks that question my claim. Understandably so because of the confusion surrounding this fact. If it were me, I would also wonder. The month before, I walked with a walking stick, and it was pretty evident that I needed it for assistance. A month later, I have no walking stick in sight. Today you may see me wearing spectacles. A month later, no spectacles.

To better explain this fact, I will refer to three people. 1) Next to where we live is a shopping centre. I know the security guard there has very many, MANY, questions. He has never expressed them but his facial expression when he sees me does. I have never had a conversation with the guy to explain the medical challenge I am dealing with. I will do one of these fine days. 2) A person who knows about my medical condition and has seen the change is the gym owner where I used to work out before I got my home gym. While I was a member of his gym, he once found me on the rowing machine. He was so impressed that I still had a dedication to going to the gym despite everything, while he spends most of his time telling able-bodied individuals to go to the gym. The irony. I hope my presence in the gym will encourage someone someday. 3) The guys I will forever admire are from where I undertake my physiotherapy. These guys knew about MS. They knew of its path and decided to take me on board and beat the condition together. Before joining Range of Motion (R.O.M.), one had to undergo a physical assessment. With the trainer who is assigned your case, you have to sit down and plan your exercises with a goal in sight. After my initial assessment, the trainer was honest enough to tell me that my physical position was terrible, BUT with constant training, it could improve. I was sold. I started with them in 2016, and I still attend the same gym to date. I've had three different physiotherapists over the years, and they have all been fantastic. Three, because life happens.

Coming to terms with these simple life changes was a challenge. Using a scooter at work was a bit hard to bear, especially having to explain my health position to the many retailers in the mall who suddenly noticed me using a scooter that I was not using a few weeks back. In retrospect, I am sure my presence at my workplace increased my understanding of MS. 'How?' You may ask. I was asked many questions by many people, and I hate the answer 'I don't know', so I did a lot of reading to answer any such questions resulting in a better understanding of the condition. My workmates were a solid backbone for my journey because we were in the same boat of discovering what MS was. Apart from my manager, who had an idea of what MS was, we were all clueless.

Working in security, you never knew what was around the corner. One minute you seem to be enjoying a relaxing shift, next thing, someone is on the radio asking for assistance. Today you are dealing with a drunk individual; tomorrow, a drug-affected person decides to be a problem. It was a place where a situation went from 0 to 100 in no time. We had to be on our toes. Always. My workmates were as worried as I was when we got a better understanding of MS. We had our way of showing concern and of helping. Someone will not come up to you and ask you if you need any help, but they will go beyond their duties to make sure your work is as simple as it can be. After my diagnosis, I spent most of my shift in the office writing up reports, checking the CCTV, answering the office phone (which at times would ring more than a phone line in a call centre), signing in contractors, and other office duties. Sometimes I wondered how we survived all that when I was on the entire 12-hour shift roster. I would write up a certain number of reports, but the next day when I start my shift again, I would notice that the number of reports in the system had increased. I never questioned this because it was something I would expect from our team.

Another reality that would be a hard pill to swallow was to do with parking. Yes. It seems petty, but it was definitely not a walk in the park. When I got diagnosed, and before I stayed away from driving for a while, I knew I could apply for an ACROD parking permit. These permits are explicitly for persons with a disability who have difficulty with mobility. In most establishments, the parking spots closest to the entrance are reserved for holders of this parking permit, and fines could be enforced if someone parks in these spots without displaying the permit. Immediately after diagnosis, I could not bring myself to apply for this permit. I knew I needed it, but in my mind, it meant that I was going to be considered a 'disabled' person, and I was somewhat ashamed. Yep. I said it. I knew that having that permit would cement a reality I did not want. In hindsight, I would have gotten it though I intended to work on overcoming the disabling element.

Having a better understanding of MS and other disabling conditions, diseases, and incidents, I am now ashamed of being embarrassed then. Most people living with a disability are the way they are not because they 'wanted' to be that way. They will change their jobs, environments, diets, and much more to accommodate the reality they have found themselves in. I have said 'most' because, believe it or not, I once heard that there are people out there who intentionally amputate their limbs so that they can be considered disabled. I kid you not. It is a condition (Google this. Please. I did, and I was as shocked as you are right now). Slowly but surely, I started warming up to the fact that reality as I knew it, or as I had planned it, had changed. In my late teenage years, I believed in planning my life, and I guess I did not expect it to have a drastic change that would alter my whole plan. Study, start a family, and live happily ever after. That was the plan. It was a fairy tale plan. Up until MS happened. Then I understood what 'planning for a rainy day' really meant. I went to therapy to help me digest the news. I knew I had to change my view of MS and disability to live with myself.

I am very blessed to be in a country with a deeper understanding of MS. I always watch the morning news because I am always amazed at how many medical discoveries are made every day. Medications to eliminate MS are yet to make the morning news, but it is always encouraging to see researchers doing what they do best. Whether it be Alzheimer's, cancer, back pain, whatever breakthrough. By going through what I had gone through when I was diagnosed with MS, I can say that the sympathy and understanding that sometimes we do not know which card will be dealt to us in life has increased, and we are many in this boat of wondering how we ended up with a disease or condition.

Acceptance of reality does not mean you will be bound by what it is you are accepting. It is accepting that one's reality has changed, but you can ensure that that change does not take you down. I have stated before that I am Christian by creed, and religion has played a significant role in helping me accept that there has been a change, but with God by my side, MS will not take me down. Thinking back at the time I received the diagnosis, the thought that God was punishing me for something I had done had crossed my mind. Hey, I am trying to be honest here. This was until I read the book of Job in the Bible. Ok, for those who are unfamiliar with the book of Job, I got your back. Here we go. Disclaimer, this is a very brief summary of the book of Job in the Bible. NOT an overview of the Bible.

In the Bible, close to the middle, you will find the book of

Job. Job was a man of God who hated evil. He had a loving and large family, and he had a lot of property. Satan, wanting to prove that Job was a loyal servant of God because he was 'pampered' by God, wanted to test Job's faith by taking away all he had and see how fast Job would curse the Lord. God, having faith in Job, agreed. He would not interfere with Satan's plans as long as Satan did not kill Job. Job lost his family members, property, and finally, his health was affected, but not once did Job say anything against God. After Satan had done his worst and Job stuck to his faith, God rewarded Job by making it possible to replace all he had lost. Satan lost. Summary done.

As human beings, it is not suffering as such that troubles us. It is undeserved suffering that troubles us. We are so used to the existence of an action and a reaction that we try to justify or understand a problem. We find it difficult when we find no reason or explanation.

CHAPTER 5

STEM CELL TREATMENT 1.0.1

Stem Cell Treatment is one of the decisions I made that would help change the course of MS. I had heard of this form of treatment before as I was discovering information regarding MS and the treatments available (for clarity purposes, there is no 'treatment' for MS. Most procedures tend to somewhat stop and/or delay MS activity). Immediately after I received the diagnosis, I believed that treating MS was as simple as taking the right pill, and in no time, I would be back to the former me. Now, let us just say I understand the complexities surrounding my health predicament.

I had lost hope in trying to find a solution or something that would not make MS look like the end of the world. I had tried many things, and I had not gotten the results I wanted. I was getting tired of trying. MS seemed more complicated than I thought. It was now sinking in that this was no flu. Then my mom happened to mention stem cell treatment in one of our many conversations. She had seen something on T.V, and she thought I had not come across it. Her mentioning it had reignited my search and my want for an answer. I knew I would not rest until I had exhausted all the avenues available to me, and this was the final one. The 'do or die' step.

I now shifted all my research efforts to stem cell treatments and who did them. At least I knew that it was provided by specific hospitals, and my main task was to identify the providers and narrow them down to my preferred provider. The simplest thing I can compare it with is choosing which school to go to. Education is offered in all schools, but something will stand out in one school to make you desire to attend a specific school. Knowing that MS was a headache to many in the field, choosing was not going to be easy. The stakes, too, were high. While researching stem cell treatments, I discovered that the procedure COULD sometimes go south, and by south, I mean beyond 'south'. I could either be paralysed or, drum roll please, lose my life. I knew I was playing with the heavy rollers now. I had to pick the guys I thought would not kill me or land me in a wheelchair.

Stem cell treatment for MS was not offered in Australia; that was my first NO. Other countries were dropped as fast. My final five were America, China, Russia, Ukraine, and Israel. The treatment I was after was offered in institutions in these five countries, but I still had the task of turning five into one. I slept on this issue for a week or so. Then I was back to elimination. America was too expensive, out. Russia and Ukraine, being a fun of international politics, this region was to be avoided for personal security reasons. I was left with China and Israel. I had used 'personal security' to eliminate Russia and Ukraine, and I would not use it again. Confidence. That was the smoking gun. I was in communication with institutions in both these countries, and I intended to choose a winner based on the level of confidence in the procedure. If a hospital in these two countries showed more confidence than the other, that was the winner. For those wondering where Jane was when all this was taking place, Jane knew I would cover all the bases when I heard my life would be on the line, and she told me to make a choice, and she would be standing next to me when I made the decision. I am sure she noticed when I was deep in thought that I was only thinking of where to go for the procedure. I told her when I was stuck, and she helped me view a situation from a different point. She was and still is my 'voice of reason'.

Then one day, during one of my calls to the hospital in Israel, the person on the other end of the line said something that would make my decision easy. He was like, 'You know this procedure MIGHT FAIL'. After that call, I called the hospital in China, and the person on the line was like, 'You might have doubts in your mind, but you will witness the positives even before you leave for home'. That was the conversation that won Beijing Puhua Hospital the deal. China it was.

When Jane got home after work, I informed her of my decision, and she was delighted that a decision had been made. Finally.

It was a long time coming, but it had been done. We were going to China. Stage one, done.

Now to get there. I had asked about the financial bill that would need to be paid for the procedure. It was precisely US$32,300.00. Ok, now the task was how to get the money. I had graduated from university close to two months before, and I did not get the chance to make a bit of money to cater to the whole procedure's finances. I was on a medication that cost an arm and a leg every twenty-eight days. I had neurology appointments to attend to, I had to rely on a taxi for my movements as I was not driving, I had been made re-dundant earlier in the year. In summary, finances were a whole new challenge. Next to impossible is an understatement.

Allow me to try and address some Kenyan visitation habits for non-Kenyans in the house. 1) There are no protocols. This is to say, we kind of 'pop in'. I will ' pop in' if I am in an area close to a friend's house. We call ahead to know if someone is home first, though. 2) When someone 'pops in', our culture dictates we offer the visitor something to drink and if it is close to mealtime, guess what? You will be included. 3) Because of 1) & 2), we do not visit empty-handed. People bring fruits and several other food-related stuff. 4) BYO for drinkers. If you visit most of our friends' houses, you will find an assortment of alcoholic drinks. The dweller might not be someone who drinks alcohol, but their friends do. Most tend to come with their favourite drink and do not leave with it because next time they decide to 'pop in' and you are a distance away from the bottle shop, they will most likely find that bottle of whiskey, or whatever it is they came with, waiting for them.

One evening we were discussing funding options available when Jane's cousin, who lived a five-minute walk away, 'popped in'. Our close friends Sam and Brian had come over for dinner. We decided to hear what options were open from the whole group. 'Crowdfund it', Jane's cousin said. She explained the working of having a GoFundMe page, and we agreed it was a good plan. We also agreed to set up a committee to spearhead the campaign. I spoke to my brother in Kenya, and he agreed to coordinate fundraising efforts there. The next few weeks were spent organising this. The committee also agreed to hold a BBQ as a fundraising activity. Point to self, never underestimate the power of the masses. I say this because we discussed carrying out a fundraiser in December, as everybody was prepping for Christmas and New Year. I had a wonderful committee for support. All preparation was finalised, and the campaign was launched. A target of US$20,000 was set for the GoFundMe, and US$10,000 was set for the fundraiser in Kenya. We were advertising the GoFundMe page daily, and the response was terrific.

We have a Swahili saying, 'kidogo kidogo hujaza kibaba'. I will not directly translate this because the risk of the meaning being lost in translation is high. Simply put, it means that 'a lot of small steps can make a big difference'. In fundraising efforts, this statement is critical because the thinking is, 'instead of a few people giving a lot, it is much easier for a lot of people to contribute a small amount. $5, $50, or $100. Nothing was too small. Every day we saw that target getting closer and closer. I received messages from everywhere. Well-wishers, others inquiring why I was running a fundraising campaign, people I know, people I might never meet, in short, my faith in humanity was cemented. One message I received was from a lady from Poland. POLAND. The lady stated that she did not know me in this message, but she had read the GoFundMe story and wanted to contribute. She wished me success with the campaign and my treatment. If someone is wondering why I post my accomplishments online every once in a while, this is one of the reasons, i.e., so that individuals like this lady would know that I am faring well.

By the first week of 2016, the target had been achieved. One month, countless adverts, 174 donations, a BBQ fundraising event, monies received through bank transfers, a total of $20,330 was reached. God is good. I called my brother back home with the news and to check how the campaign there was going, and he summarised it in five words, 'you are going to China'. I was overjoyed. 'This is happening for real' I said to myself. No more maybes or what-ifs. It was a go for China.

The next day I went to apply for visas for Jane and me and emailed the hospital to inform them that I was going. Stage two, done.

CHAPTER 6

DESTINATION CHINA

Neither Jane nor I had been to China before, so we were learning on the go. The good thing was that I was in the company of the best person to do it with. Wing it till you win it. (Yes, people expect me to say that because she is my wife, but she was and still is the best person to have been with for real.)

To say the truth, the only thing I remember about our trip to China is that we were flying with Singapore Airlines. My whole trip was a moment of reflection. I knew lumbar punctures were involved (Yes, plural). How fast it would take to be able to run after the treatment? What I would do? I thought about a lot of things. Unfortunately, I had not considered recovery time and all the work

I had to dedicate to it. Now, I know better.

Our first challenge was to do with Chinese immigration. Yes, at the airport. My passport, thanks to my lovely wife who had decided to give it a spin in the washing machine (this is a 'she said, he said' story for another day), had suffered water damage. I had not gone home since I went to Australia as a student four years before to get a new one. Unintentionally so. Chinese immigration had had people go there with fake passports before, and mine did not look so pretty not to raise a few eyebrows. Jane and I were sent to an office as the immigration officer verified the travel document. Our saving grace, though we were not told so, I believe was Jane's Australian passport. We could see my passport being taken all around as they verified its authenticity. The immigration officer came back and handed me my passport. We were cleared to enter. The hospital had organised for an airport pickup, which made it easy considering the airport was forty-five minutes from the hospital. We had gone during winter, and the cold was on a different level. Thank God the car had a heater. Massive buildings, most of them were apartments blocks. And very many vehicles. Small. Many small cars.

We got to the hospital where we were shown our room, ok my bed and Jane's sofa bed. The room was self-contained with a kitchenette in one of the corners; it had everything one could need in a hospital room. We were also shown the main kitchen area if we needed a more significant cooking space. After a brief walkthrough of the hospital, we were shown the theatre, which I would visit thrice when in hospital, and the physiotherapy rooms. There was a restaurant within the hospital walls for the days we just did not fancy cooking, and that was it. Jane was shown where to catch a cab and all, but that was that. I say Jane because I could not leave the hospital for the next three weeks. My immunity was expected to be compromised with the many medical procedures planned, and it was best I stayed in the hospital.

First on our busy schedule was for Jane and I to take 'flu prevention medication. This was only day one, and we knew the hospital was extremely careful that flu comes nowhere around the patients. After taking the tablets, we were relaxing in the room when the door swung open, and the doctors who would administer the stem cells came in. They introduced themselves and explained the procedure even though they had done it before, during my countless phone calls. This allowed us to ask any questions we had, which were quite a number. After roughly an hour, the doctors were out. At least we now knew we were in safe hands. In summary, I was to have three procedures done on me, all to do with a lumbar puncture. One every week. Also, for the duration of my hospital stay, I was to have acupuncture, a few Chinese medicine tablets, and a massage and physiotherapy daily. Yes, daily. In case anyone is thinking of going there, Beijing Puhua International Hospital. Google it. They will give you more information when you contact them. The information above is a summary of the summary.

Then there was a change of shift by the nurses. To date, I never understood why they all came at the same time. And they all had some 'fake' English names. Back to where I was, our room was flooded by around twelve to fifteen nurses. FLOODED. It was clear not all of them were good in English but then again, I was not there to see whether they could speak it. The doctors were good at it; that is good enough for me. Then the theatrics began. This next part was unbelievably funny. Some of the nurses came up to the bed and started poking me, saying, 'you too big, you too big'. I was in utter shock, and when I looked at Jane for support, she was inches from the floor laughing. I think she laughed so hard she even shed a tear or two. Well, after the nurses absorbed the size of the new guy, the head nurse explained that they had to up the dosage of the medication because it had been measured for a person of a smaller body size. In my mind, I was thinking of the many family members and friends I had who were bigger than I was. I am approximately 90 kg, and the dosage was for someone on the 60 – 70 kg mark. If you put it that way, it kind of makes sense.

We got to China on a Friday and thought all those medications and procedures would begin on Monday. Nope. The very same day. We were time-bound because the Chinese New Year was scheduled for the 8th of Feb 2016. We had approximately two weeks to experience its effect.

The next day Jane decided she would go out and see the neighbourhood as she bought a few items for our 'home' away from home. She went out and came back with bags of groceries, an assortment of beef, pork, and chicken meat, and a pocketknife. Yes, POCKETKNIFE. Luckily our 'go-to person' was making her rounds, and we asked about the pocketknife when she came in for a welfare check. Apparently, sometime in the past, some maniac decided to chop up a few people with knives that were on display for sale. Since then, a person needed a police certificate to buy a knife or something on those lines. Oh, and not all persons sell them. Purchasing a knife was like buying a gun. Yeah, it shocked us too. Well, we were now proud owners of a 1.5-inch blade pocketknife to do most of our slicing of vegetables and meats and everything that needs cutting.

Week one was ok. Snow was falling. I could not touch it, but we could see it fall through the window. The hospital premises were warm, but I could see the people outside were cold. Again, through the window. In short, I experienced a white winter through the window. That sounds about right. The day I was dreading came. Wednesday, January 20th. The first of three lumbar punctures.

The doctor carrying out the procedure came and explained it to us again. I would be transferred to a theatre bed, rolled into theatre, have to position myself to the surgeon's specific instructions, and have the operation done while awake but pumped with heavy pain medication. I would be back to the room, transferred to my bed where I would be expected to remain for six hours. 'Six?' I asked. 'Yes. Six,' she replied. I thought of looking at Jane for her negotiating skills to kick in, but this was the doctor telling us. No negotiation could change this, so I did not even try. The doctor left and let us digest what she had said. An hour and a half later, a nurse came and ushered me to another bed. He wheeled it to the theatre, where I found a team of surgeons waiting. I was asked to lie in the foetal position, and the last sensation I had on my back was of the doctor trying to feel the discs in my spine to know which entry point to use. I was lucky they numbed the spot before inserting the injection.

'How big was the injection?' you may ask. Your guess is as good as mine. I remember during my first lumbar puncture, the doctor who was carrying out the procedure, for the sake of making me feel relaxed, decided to start a conversation. He informed me that I could view what he was doing with the help of a camera that takes the video of what is happening inside my spine. 'Why would I want to do that?' was my question to him. I did not want to sound rude but seeing a needle stuck into my spine was too much for me. I apologised when he had finished, and explained injections/needles are a no-no for me.

Anyway, before I knew it, I was done. It took fifteen to twenty minutes. I was wheeled back to the room where Jane was curious about how it went. I could not get up to get to my bed. I was not allowed to. Some nurses were there to help transfer me to my bed. They were not Chinese. Once on my bed, I was reminded not to get up. If I needed to pee, they gave me a container to pee in. Number two was the only reason I could get up and commenced my six hours. Jane decided to go and explore Beijing that day.

Another point to note is that we had a TV with ninety-eight channels, ninety-six were in Chinese. To make matters worse, the two English-speaking channels repeated movies twice or thrice a day, and only they know where they picked them from. AND there was no Google. Luckily, WhatsApp was working. That day, Jane realised the language barrier was real because if you do not know Chinese, you are screwed. Let us say not much 'shopping' was done that day. It was also a day that Jane felt the wrath of winter.

To summarise the incident, she wanted to head back to the hospital, and unfortunately, most taxis refused to take her to the location she provided. She was able to get a rickshaw, and the traffic she saw on her way back explained why no taxi wanted to ply the route. To answer a question I think you might have about this experience, the hospital staff had given Jane a card indicating the hospital's location. This is what she showed taxi drivers. The 'no' was not hard to grasp, even in Chinese. Some shook their heads to indicate 'NO' while others simply drove off. The relief on Jane's face when she got back was visible. That night we tasked ourselves to make a list of what we needed, and we sent the item name in English to our family back in Australia, who looked up the Chinese word on Google and sent it to us via WhatsApp. It was a lengthy task, but it was the only way. This translation route was repeated for most of our stay.

Before I forget another fact about China, they have nil, if not very minimal, respect for personal space. One day Jane was busy oiling herself after having a bath when a female nurse walked into the room. Courtesy dictates she apologises, leaves the room, and probably comes back a bit later when Jane is done. Nope. She just gave Jane a five-second stare and turned, looked at me and gave me my meds, asked if I felt ok, and she left. For a few seconds, Jane and I were staring at the door, wondering, 'What on earth just happened?' We used to lock the door when one of us went to the shower from then on. If a nurse is supposed to attend the room and finds it locked, one expects them to continue with their rounds and come back a bit later. Nooo. The nurses used to wait at the door until it was opened. Five seconds later, five minutes later. Take a pick.

When I was not going to the theatre, we tried to find an activity for occupying our time within our room. We had a deck of cards with us, which kept us entertained. Or we saw a repeat of a movie we saw before, courtesy of the channel director. I think what made our stay positive was knowing what had taken us there. There was also the procedural acupuncture, massage, and physio. Then, it was a challenge to get out of bed, let alone walk to the physio area. I was tired after all of this. DAILY. I wished time would fly but at the same time dreaded the two lumbar punctures remaining.

Then my 'not' favourite day was upon us once again. Again, I made sure my bowels were as empty as possible, and the last bit of pee in me was out. The nurse doing the transfer came, I changed beds, and before I knew it, I was positioning myself in the usual foetal position in the theatre. We all expected the same 'quick and eventless' procedure. Expected. Again, the surgeon was feeling my spinal-disc positioning, and she believed that a change from the location she injected before was a sure thing. She explained this to me before going ahead. Then I understood why they needed patients awake for the procedure. I felt a sharp pain go down my leg to my toe and back again onto the leg. I think my back tensed up, and the surgeon knew something was not ok. Calmly she asked what I felt, and I did my best to explain the sensation to her. She then decided not to go ahead with the procedure from that area. She did a quick examination on the surrounding discs, and because the place she had injected last time had healed up fine, she decided to use it again. Instead of twenty minutes, the procedure lasted around forty-five minutes. 'Done', she said. I was so relieved it was over. Soon I was being wheeled back to our room.

When the door flung open, I could see the relief on Jane's face. Something on my face told her the procedure was not like the first one. I was transferred to my bed, and immediately after the nurses left the room, Jane asked if I was ok. I told her of my experience that day, and we thanked God it was over. To date, remembering that day gives me chills. I believe if the surgeon went ahead with their initial plan, we would be speaking a different story today. Either I would be writing this while seated in a wheelchair, or I would not be writing this at all and being referred to in the past tense. That day Jane cancelled her day's plans and sat by the bed for the whole six hours. At some point, I dozed off, and when I woke up, I could feel Jane's warm hand on mine. I so love this woman.

The days were basically the same. Repeat movies, card games, and just chat the night away. Then we started noticing a decrease in staff members. It was a noticeable number. I am not talking about one or two. No. Like half of the hospital staff members. We asked about this, and we were told that most staff members came from different parts of China and had traveled home for the Chinese New Year. The doctors and surgeons were all around, but most other staff members had travelled home. A good example was during the physio sessions, the number of staff members was almost double that of patients. Now, the ratio was 1:1.

That weekend I reminded Jane of something we had to do. After some time, it hit us. I had remembered something we had planned a couple of days back. 'What's big about that?' you may ask. I had REMEMBERED something. I never remembered anything. Since my diagnosis, my memory had gone out of the window. Well, not anymore. I could not wait to see the doctor on Monday. This joy made the weekend go faster, and before we knew it, our final week commenced. The doctor came for her rounds to find me waiting with the news. She came into the room, and I semi-yelled, 'I remembered something.' She looked at me and asked, 'aaand'? 'No. I remembered something', I repeated. I looked at her with a big smile. She was trying to figure out what it was that I had remembered and why it made me so happy. Then it hit home. 'Your memory' she said. Now we were clearly on the same page. You could see the joy in her. 'You remembered something' she also kind of semi-yelled. I looked at Jane, who was just smiling as she looked at the doctor and I, enjoying the moment. It was a very precious moment.

Slowly that week, I started going to the kitchen more to prepare meals. I had missed the kitchen. That is when I noticed that my fatigue levels had dropped. After my physio, I was usually drained, and the only thing I wanted then was to sleep. Not anymore. I felt more alive now, and despite the physio, I slept less. (This has greatly improved to where I'm now back to my five-hour sleep pattern). Apart from these improvements, our last week went ok. My third and final lumbar puncture went as eventless as the first, and it was time to go. We left the hospital, and having seen the traffic chaos of Beijing, we booked a hotel close to the airport. I had adjusted well to the treatment, and we were given medication to take for the next few months. We were given more medication against the flu as we left to feel the chill of the winter. There was no need for another appointment with the hospital.

We were impressed. The hospital had predicted three weeks, and in three weeks, we were gone. Because of the winter, not much roaming around was done, but a lot had been witnessed. Through the windows.

CHAPTER 7

ROUND 2

I thought the battle was over, but I realised I had not factored recovery in my plan. I thought after my treatment, everything would go back to the way it was, and that would be the end. WRONG. We got back, and I made appointments with the doctors I saw for us to be on the same page. Not that I had an army of doctors. The days I would go to the hospital were when I saw other doctors, but I had two primary doctors. Thank God they were in constant communication regarding my case, or else I would be forced to repeat myself every time I had an appointment. This appointment was to first explain my month-long absence and know what way forward would be expected.

For precautionary purposes, the neurologist I used to see, Dr. G, had advised I stop taking the medication I was on back in November 2015. This was after trying to talk me out of it. 'Try' being the main word here. I used to pose specific questions via email to him. It got to a point where Dr. G was on 'damage control'. He knew I would go through with it, so his advice was around what I could do to improve my position for the time when I decided to go through with it. In a way, I felt pity for Dr. G because he now had an unexpected patient who was extremely stubborn. If I decide on something, be sure I will go through with it. Deciding whether or not to go through with a plan was where most deliberations in my mind took place. As for stem cell treatment, doctors in Australia do not recommend it as a treatment option, and neither did Dr. G. After I got back from China, I gave Dr. G a call, and not to his surprise, I had gone through with the stem cell treatment. He advised that I would no longer be his patient, but he had forwarded my case to Dr. B, who had offered his opinion during my diagnosis. Dr. B was also knowledgeable about post-stem cell treatment. Who knew? Anyway, I would now be seeing Dr. B. I thought I was done, but God had another surprise in store. In summary, as much as stem cells had helped by eliminating some of the effects of MS, it had not addressed the root cause of the problem. The only difference now, that was not there before, is that I knew what to expect.

I stayed away from medication for close to a year until I felt something was not right. Unlike before, I did not delay arranging an appointment to see my GP. I saw Dr. B, who carried out some tests that were not unfamiliar to me, and I was sad to hear that MS had found its way into my system again. Not the news you would want to hear after months of no medication, our China experience, and for the many people who had stood by me encouraging me to win this fight. But that was the sad reality. The doctor ordered me to start four-weekly infusions, and he would be seeing me twice a year. A second-round would have taken me down but my knowledge, though minimal about MS, encouraged me to keep fighting. In late 2018, I went in for an appointment with Dr. B who moved my medication rotation to six-weekly from every twenty-eight days. All the physiotherapy and exercise had started showing very positive results. He extended it, and I'm praying that I continue on the same trajectory and have it stretched even further. In the end, I pray that my scans are a miracle waiting to happen and that researchers find a cure for MS. Nobody should face this condition.

As I mentioned before, Multiple Sclerosis Society of Western Australia (MSWA) had been very supportive since I received the diagnosis. An MSWA nurse is the one who paid Jane and I a visit to explain what MS was, an MSWA counsellor arranged appointments with me to tackle the mental health side of the diagnosis, a different MSWA counsellor spoke to Jane and I on the stress that such a diagnosis can bring to a relationship, an MSWA physiotherapist helped me tackle the physical strain that MS had introduced in my life. In return, I support MSWA activities by volunteering to assist where possible. Most of these events are held annually. If you hear of one, please pop in and ask of ways you can help if your participation is impossible. Last year, 2020, for the first time, I was able to ride a bike in one of the MSWA events, the Ocean Bike Ride. After all my training, I finished the 10 km bike ride. Because of my balance challenge, I looked for a tricycle to make this dream a reality.

An injury was constantly on my mind. I had to be honest with myself that a fall, once in a while, was somewhat expected considering. Not always, but sometimes. Having balance challenges, I developed a habit of knowing my surroundings well to a point where if I were to lose my balance, where and what I would turn to for more support. If I was walking into a building, I would endeavour to walk next to someone I knew had the strength to 'rescue' me if things were to go south. All this with a walking stick in my hand. Who said men can't multitask?

One specific night we had gone to a friend's party, and as I walked into the house, I miscalculated the height of the step from the garage, where we were sitting. I was going in briefly, then my balance failed. One minute I was walking into a house; the next minute, I could tell you the brand of shoe the guy in front of me was wearing. (To show how much I had pre-planned for a fall, I knew which side was best to fall on. My right shoulder side was safer. It was probably because it was the one side I had never had any injury and had done a lot of weight training). I landed on my right shoulder. Unfortunately, any fall of a 90 kg person would cause a bit of tear. I had the onsite first aid massage, but I visited my GP the following day. I was sure I had damaged something. The GP gave me some pain medication and sent me to see a physiotherapist.

I visited the physiotherapist at one of the local hospitals. We mapped out a plan on what to do and when my goals will be achieved. During my subsequent visits, we spoke of some of the challenges I had faced, from judgemental physiotherapists to hearing some misunderstood beliefs on MS. She believed I should give lectures to physiotherapy students and tell my story because she noticed I was ready to put across my side of the story and who better to give it than someone who has had to visit several physiotherapists. I focus on students because if you ask me, their thinking has not been clouded by opinions on what to expect from a client with a specific condition or disease. Not that experience does not matter. It does. However, I believe that students are best to learn on how to rid their minds of any beliefs that would cloud their future practices.

The one thing that is not affected by MS is someone's brain. Most warriors might be suffering from mental health wellbeing issues because of what they suffer or have experienced in their fight. As for my case, I had survived depression because it was hard to comprehend how one night could alter what I thought was going to be my future. Knowing my brain function had not been affected, I decided to pursue a course and be a qualified travel agent. Now that I could not practice law, I decided to go into a career that I loved, and I love travel. In 2017, I undertook a one-year-long course, and in 2018, I started a business, Bara Travel & Tours.

On 25th September 2019, my wife and I were blessed with a baby boy. Anyway, a son, a wife, a business, my health, let us just say my time is not an individual thing anymore. I have people who rely on me. Me staying strong is not an option. I have to stay strong. For how long? Only God can answer that.

CHAPTER 8

IT IS NOT OVER UNTIL THE FAT LADY SINGS

2020 came with its own challenge and my second retirement from the workforce because I had to close down my business. The world was facing a global pandemic that would claim many lives. Living in Western Australia, the state government was stringent on who could come into the state. That, I believe, is what saved many lives here. Knowing that only part of our family was in Australia was pretty hard. What made it even more real was the fact that every time I went to the hospital to receive my six-weekly infusion, I passed in front of the temporary Covid tent that had been built at the hospital. Every six weeks. It was just a reminder that the world still had a pandemic it was dealing with. Thinking about the pandemic brought with it a memory of a time when I was unsure of what ailed me. Covid was a health scare with no cure. To make matters worse, it was predicted to be a big problem for people who have underlying health conditions. Wow, as if I did not have enough on my mind already. Anyway, most of us are waiting for the medical researchers to figure MS out. Unfortunately, not everyone shared this sentiment since vaccines against a global pandemic were in circulation in just over a year. That aside, I called my GP, the neurologist, and MSWA to find out the effects of this vaccine on me, who goes for an infusion every couple of weeks. Get this, they did not know. Yep. They found a nice way of telling me to have the vaccine, and if I react to it, 'IF', then they would know there is a clash of both medications. Anyway, I plan to have my dose mainly because of Jane's job description and make sure Chege will not lose his father because I chose to believe conspiracy theories.

I am now an Australian citizen. This does not mean much to some people, but it does to me. To bring you into my world, I received a diagnosis when I was still on my student visa. From a student visa, I had to move to a graduate visa after graduating. After that, I had to go onto a bridging visa, then a partner visa, and finally became a citizen. In total, seven years. It took three to four years to transition from a graduate visa to a permanent resident, which was the longest. In defense of the Australian immigration department, my visa process had changed. If I was not ill, then I believe it would have taken a shorter time.

In 2014, I had had a very long talk with my mom regarding my citizenship. My initial plan was to finish my studies and go back home. My greatest challenge then was convincing Jane on what was next. That was the initial plan. When I got sick, it changed. I firmly believe that researchers in Australia will unlock the secret behind MS. Truth be told, I do not care who cracks this condition first. I just wait for the day they do. Having said that, I explained to my mom how my plan had changed. Doctors in Australia had a better understanding of the condition that I was facing. It was not a foreign case to them. It's not that doctors in Kenya do not know about it, but chances were higher for doctors in Australia to have come across a patient with MS than it was for a doctor in Kenya to deal with such a case. Coming from Kenya and knowing how life there is, let us just say my belief in the government processes there left a lot to be desired. That is the government. The health department, hmmm…

Then comes the cost of medication. In 2014, the drug I was on cost me around $1500 every twenty-eight days. You see all the talk on the advantages of having health insurance; it is accurate. My out-of-pocket was about $200. My health insurance took care of the rest. I would have for sure drowned in debt if I never had health insurance. When my visa changed in 2016, I changed the hospital I received the infusion. My sister had accompanied me for my first appointment at the new location. She told me that she would pay for the medication. We got to the hospital pharmacy where we purchased the medicine, and they told her it would cost $46 or something ridiculous like that. My sister was in the process of transferring funds into one account so that she could make the payment. I almost died of shock. WHAT? The medicine had moved from $1500 a dose to less than $50. I am not done; when I became a permanent resident, it changed to $6. You heard me right.

$6 (six dollars).

So, whoever decides to question the government's position to make certain drugs cheaper, don't. It lightens the load. I am usually in the queue at the hospital pharmacy, and I do not think I can count the number of people I have come across who benefit from such schemes. Cancer patients especially because they must take several drugs, some daily.

I am still going for my physio sessions. Twice a week now. I have received a lot of encouragement from the Range of Motion family, and in 2022, I will apply to be in a Crossfit competition. There is a new category of individuals who suffer from neuromuscular challenges that I want to participate in. This year, 2021, I will participate in the 30 km bike ride. I am training for it, do not worry. It will be a challenge, but I will not give it a chance to win. Jane and Mr. Chege will participate in the 10 km family ride.

I am studying for a Master of Counselling degree, and I will graduate in 2022. You would think I know everything after such a challenging couple of years. I am learning so much that I never knew, and I hope that the knowledge I get and my experience with difficult situations will benefit someone else someday. I must admit the walk has been challenging, and I might have doubted if I would make it through. However, I made it through, and I am sure we all have this same 'will' to make it. All we must do is dig deep and fish out the will to fight.

Regarding finding some form of employment, I thought it was a myth that people living with a disability will try and, in most cases, will not find work. I take that thought back. After the diagnosis, I was made redundant in 2015. I applied for jobs. Unsuccessfully. This was one of the reasons why I started my own business. I think I was on the 100-150 job applications. One day I went to meet a lady who was meant to assist me in finding a job (I will not specify which office) who commented that 'you will not be able to find employment especially with your condition because if someone is to employ you, they would have to make a lot of changes to their policies, procedures, insurance and such, which is costly.' I don't think she intended to say that aloud, but it was out. This explained many things, but after my business went under because of Covid-19 in 2020, I continued applying for jobs. By mid-2021, I believe I was around the 300-350 mark.

There was a time I started making a joke that people seemed to be afraid of my walking stick but had no way of informing me. Then out of the blue, the Bureau of Statistics called me to arrange a job interview. I finally got a job. God is good. After six years of applying. I am approximating because, truth be told, knowing the exact number was becoming quite demoralising, and I had decided to stop counting anymore when I got to around thirty applications. Oh, and by my 350 mark, I think I have seriously short-changed myself. The actual number is about 1,500 applications. My greatest encouragement on this front was my religion and my mom. As a Christian, I never for a second thought that my prayers for a job were in vain, and my mom made sure I never forgot that. My siblings and I witnessed our parents investing their time and money in many ventures when growing up. This push never stopped after my dad died. Knowing she would now be running solo, my mom has always been up to something to date.

If I ever call my mom and when I ask what she is up to and she tells me 'Nothing', alarm bells start going off because I know she is no longer planning. Whatever it is, it is going down. This is one of the reasons why I never stopped applying for jobs despite receiving countless apology emails. Because when I got that call in 2021 of a job offer, I called my mom to tell her the great news, and she could only afford a few words, 'what did I tell you?' That is the reply she gave me. Mentioning it so casually should not be taken to mean it was easy. I was halfway filling up an application many times, and a voice inside my head would encourage me to stop because of the number of rejection notifications I had received, but the Christian in me did not want to hear it. I would go ahead and apply.

As a parting shot, I would like to thank everyone who made my journey possible. Yes, it might have had its ups and downs, but interesting is an understatement. God, Jane, Baby Chege (you have an amazing mum), my family and friends, my doctors, nurses, and other professionals in all the many hospitals I have visited over the years, MSWA, MS Australia, MS Kenya, Westfield, my former workmates, contributors to my campaign to go to China, Beijing Puhua Hospital, R.O.M team, GetFitForLife gym, Your Travel & Cruise Pty, University of Western Australia alumni relations, University of Notre Dame, Edith Cowan University, and each and every individual that has contributed to making my journey as comfortable as it could be. God bless you all.